My Crazy Life: Living with MS

TANGIE ESSARY

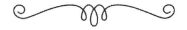

Copyright © 2022 Tangie Essary

All rights reserved.

No part of this book may be used or reproduced by any means, graphic, electronic, or mechanical, including photocopying, recording, taping, or by any information storage retrieval system without the written permission of the publisher except in the case of brief quotations embodied in critical articles and reviews.

ISBN: 9798404089301

My Crazy Life While Living with MS, LLC

First Edition 2022

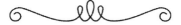

This book is dedicated to God

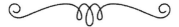

CONTENTS

	Acknowledgments	i
1	The Dresser	1
2	Missouri	6
3	Back to Oroville	12
4	The Breakup	24
5	Medication Free	36
6	Hardships	45
7	Wings	50
8	COVID	54

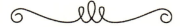

ACKNOWLEDGMENTS

*Thank you very much to
Kristi Stalder, Sarah Nelson,
Shirley McAllister and Alyse Dahlquist
for helping me get this book out.*

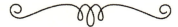

THE DRESSER

It was a chilly, cloudy day on May 26th, 1962, when my mother went into labor. I was delivered at the only hospital in the small town of Tonasket, Washington, in room 18 at 12:08 pm.

My parents—Manford and Billie Essary—were so excited to welcome the new addition to their family. My mother did not have a name picked out the moment I was born. Later, she remembered that she had been craving tangerines during labor, so she decided to name me Tangie.

My parents were young and poor at the time. They brought me home to a picker cabin where they lived while my father worked for an orchardist, Ted Thorndike, in an apple orchard.

There was no crib for me, so my mom emptied a dresser drawer and lined it with blankets to make it soft. That was my bed.

One day, while cleaning the cabin, mom shut the drawer and forgot I was still inside. When she remembered a bit later, she panicked! Opening the drawer, she was surprised to find me still asleep. It was then she realized that I was adaptive and ready to handle whatever life threw at me.

As I grew older, I started to learn how to walk. My parents gave me the nickname 'Toshy-boom-boom' because I fell down a lot! I would glare at anyone who called me that as a kid, but as an adult, I came to find that nickname cute and funny.

Soon after I started walking, my parents moved in with my grandparents on my dad's side. They lived at Whitestone, just above Tonasket. My earliest memories are from living with my grandparents. My Grandpa would come home for his lunch break, and I would hide behind the back door to scare him. He always acted scared and would smile. One day, he forgot and came through the front door instead. My grandma made him go back outside and come through the back door just so I could jump out and scare him.

This is just one of many memories that I have of living in that house. I treasure those times, from painting my grandparent's picnic table yellow with dandelions, floating my toy boats in Grandma's rinse water while she washed the dishes, and sitting on Grandma's lap while she sang the song, "I've Got a Mansion."

Of course, there were tough times that I faced while living there, too. My cousin, Tawanna, and I had chickenpox. And there was a time when my mom was making a quilt, and I wanted to climb up onto the bed with her. When she pulled me up by the arms, one of my arms dislocated from its socket. Thank goodness I don't remember the incident, but I do know that it was just one of the obstacles I had overcome during my childhood.

Unfortunately, I do remember a fight between my parents. My dad slammed the door as he left the laundry room where my mom and I were standing. My mom threw a clothes iron at my dad and hit the door, causing a triangle-shaped imprint on the door. I didn't know what that fight was about, but that memory still stuck with me.

One of my favorite memories is that my family would all gather on Sunday mornings. We would have church in my grandparent's living room, and this was when I began to learn about God.

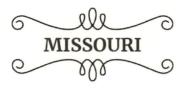

MISSOURI

When I was seven years old, my Dad, Mom, and younger sister, Tina, and I moved to Missouri.

When we arrived, I was enrolled in school. My dad's uncle Clarence was my school bus driver.

My grandmother, Lena (whom we called Lean,) was dying of lung cancer. She lived with my Uncle Clarence, Aunt Fae, and their daughters, Deborah, Della, and Carla. Grandma Lean lived with them until she had to be moved to the hospital in

Springfield. Since Uncle Clarence was my bus driver, I was able to keep up with what was going on with my grandma.

At first, we lived in a small camp trailer in my cousins' Dub and Genivie's yard. They had twin boys, Boyd and Coy, who I played with. We lived there so we could be near my grandma Lean. Shortly after that, we moved into a trailer court in Goldendale, Missouri.

One day, Mom was sitting with Grandma Lean in the hospital and arranged for Genevie to pick me up after school. For some reason, she had forgotten all about me. I sat on the front porch crying for what seemed like an hour before she remembered and came to pick me up. It was very scary because I had never been alone before and I didn't know anyone in the trailer court.

Being the new kid in school, I felt the need to be liked. When I spotted a copperhead snake coiled up on the basketball court, I grabbed a rock and threw it as hard as I could. I hit the snake square on top of its head! The snake's head flopped sideways with its mouth open, appearing to be dead. Until this day, I don't know if it was truly dead, but all of the other kids thought I did it, and that's the best part.

The summers were scorchers in Missouri. I remember running across the road to see my grandma, and it was so hot the tar came to the top of the pavement. I was always running around barefoot, and my feet would burn and blister from the hot tar sticking to them.

My great-grandma Mamie's house was next door to Dub and Genivies, so we got to see her often. Her house was very small. She collected rainwater from a barrel that sat in her front yard. She would strain the water with a cotton dish towel and use it for drinking water. There were a lot of Granddaddy Long Leg spiders on the walls in her house. Being arachnophobic, I wanted her to kill them all! She would tell me, "No, they keep the bugs down and are harmless."

Grandma Mamie chewed tobacco and had a spit can by her chair. She also had a small dog that would run out into the middle of the road, and it got run over often. My grandma would go over to the dog and pray for it, and that dog would stagger up and shake itself off. Then, to everyone's amazement, it would trot back into the yard as if nothing had happened.

Mom left me with my cousins Olen, Jeanie, and Olena while she was with Grandma Lean in the hospital.

One day, when mom came home to pick me up, she told me that Grandma had gone to Heaven. I was devastated. After a long time of crying, I got it together enough to leave. Without my grandma's existence, I felt so alone.

My parents took me to my cousins. The weeds and wildflowers in the sweltering heat smelled so good while we were catching fireflies. Putting them into a jar with my cousins Lamond and Wilda's kids Farren, Tim, Tony, Marty, and Pam. Yes, I had a lot of cousins everywhere! Family was plentiful in Missouri. My favorite thing about going to their house was when their mom would have us go in the backyard and pick blackberries. Then, she would make a great, big blackberry cobbler!

BACK TO OROVILLE

On top of losing my grandma, I found out the devastating news that my parents had separated.

Mom packed up everything up along with my sister and me, and we moved back to Oroville, Washington. We traveled on a greyhound bus and had a layover in North Dakota. We had to kill some time, so we walked around, and it was extremely cold. When we got back to Washington, we stayed with my mom's mom, Grandma

Lola, and mom's youngest siblings, Clifford and Teresa, who were near my age, and we became very close.

Fortunately, my parents were able to work through their differences, and they reconnected. Together, we all moved into a house where I spent the years from age eight through sixteen.

My father was an Evangelist part-time, and my mother was adamant about being in church every time the doors were open. I learned about God, His Word, and His instructions that He expected for us to live by. I gained my strength from His teachings, which would impact my life in a major way.

My family was comprised of musicians, and we would have a jam session going in our living room a lot of the time. My dad asked me to sing for his friends, and I grew up with a microphone in my face. I would sing with my family as we went to different churches with Dad while he preached. Years down the road, my sister—who was four and a half years younger than me—began singing and playing piano, joining the family jam session before our group fizzled out.

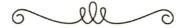

June 17th, 1975

While tossing a tennis ball across the yard with my cousin Kim, a strange feeling came over me. I began to throw the ball to the ground, unable to throw it as I was before.

Then, I started staggering around.

Kim helped me into the house, and I explained to my mother what was happening. Concerned, she called the Pastor's brother and Sister Cockrill from our church. When the symptoms continued, they came and prayed for me and advised my parents to get medical help and take me to Wenatchee, Washington.

I was in the hospital for five days with tests being run back to back. After a spinal tap, which was very painful, my mom could hear me screaming and crying from the waiting room. She had a hard time not busting into the room. Being fevered, the electroencephalogram, or EEG test to detect abnormalities of the brain, was difficult because the pins kept falling out of my head. The doctor had to keep replacing them, causing me more pain. There were

MRIs and more tests, but I was so fevered I can't remember them all.

There was a nurse that I became close to who brought me a stuffed Snoopy dog that had all the doctor's and nurse's signatures on it. Being in Wenatchee, nearly two and a half hours away from home, I didn't have people around me that I knew other than my parents. That was until Kenneth and Dorothy Felton (more cousins) who lived in Wenatchee came to see me. After the fifth day of tests and no answers, I was released to go home. The doctors were just as baffled as we were.

After two years of doctors and specialists arguing over my diagnosis and thinking that I may have had encephalitis (fever on the brain which is common in cattle,) having a sense of humor, I remember saying, "I checked my whole family tree, and there is not a Holstein in the herd."

Dr. Ranken, the neurologist at the time (who wore a bow tie, and I forgot his name all the time, so I just called him Dr. Bowtie), called my parents and told them to bring me back to Wenatchee for a consultation. I had researched my symptoms on my own during those two years, and I had come to the conclusion that I had Multiple Sclerosis. Since I'm not a doctor, I didn't say anything.

While in Dr. Rankens office, he informed my mother and me of the official diagnosis.

I did, indeed, have Multiple Sclerosis.

Even though I already knew this, hearing it from the neurologist felt like my heart dropped into my stomach because I had read what MS entailed. I had been wishing and hoping all this time that I was wrong. After all, I wasn't a doctor, but to my horror, it was real.

I had many major exacerbations from the condition. I had to learn to do things over and over again, such as writing and walking. Being so young at the age of thirteen, I didn't understand the gravity of the situation with what was really going on. I started to get better but continued to have problems off and on. Having exacerbations on my right side and then my left side, taking turns during each episode.

Later on, while I was still thirteen, my mother took me aside and told me I had a half-sister, and her name was Sherry. She was on her way here from Springfield, Missouri, and Dad was bringing her from the airport. I was so excited to have an older sister. I had always wanted one! My sister and I got into a lot of trouble together, but we had a lot of fun. Once, we were sneaking out of the downstairs window to meet with my Uncle Clifford. My dad, however, must have heard us discussing the plan through the vents because he was already standing next to the window on the lawn as soon as we climbed through. Dad made us come inside through the front door, so Mom would see us. Mom was shocked, and needless to say, she was not happy with us.

My sister Sherry and her boyfriend James took me with them across the Canadian border, only four miles away from home when we were supposed to be at the high school basketball game. We went to the bar because the legal drinking age was lower there. They let me in even though I was only 14, without checking my ID. I was shocked, but it wasn't a big deal. I wasn't really interested in drinking. After Sherry and James had their fun seeing if they could sneak me into a bar, we left. When we crossed the border and were back into the US, James dropped us off at my dad's car, parked at the basketball game we were supposed to be at. Sherry and I cruised down Main street in dad's car, hollering out the window, "What was the score?" so we would know what to say when our parents asked us.

There were two young men who came to see my dad, and they were bluegrass musicians. Their names were Fred and Tim. Fred played guitar, and Tim played the fiddle. Tim didn't stay long, but Fred became part of the family. He and I would go to church and practice music. He and I drove down to Deep Bay in Oroville, along the edge of the water. I told him we would get stuck, and he replied, "No, it will be ok." I shrugged it off. But when I opened my door on the passenger side, I could see that we were actually in the water. After trying to get out of it, Fred realized that we were stuck. We both climbed out of the driver's side door and hurried to my Aunt's house nearby. I called my mom and told her we were stuck, so she called up a friend of ours that had a 4x4 truck. He came and pulled us out.

While driving up in the mountains a few days later, we pulled over, got out, and walked around. I left Fred, mom, and my sisters and walked clumsily over to a boulder. I sat down and quietly started to panic because my right hand and arm started tingling. That was a sign of the beginning stages of an MS exacerbation. Luckily it went away.

Things were relatively quiet during the next few years. Fred ended up marrying Lisa, who was an evangelist's daughter, and I was a bridesmaid at their wedding.

Sherry went back and forth throughout the years between Missouri to my hometown in Oroville, Washington. She ended up having two boys and married a good friend of mine named Jeff. I stayed with them for a while when I left my first husband, and I slept on my sister's couch. During the Christmas holiday season, I would wake up around midnight and could not go back to sleep; my brother-in-law started smoking a joint with me when I couldn't sleep. I had experimented with marijuana before, but not consistently. It was just for fun in the beginning, and then I realized its medicinal properties and how much better I felt when I smoked it. At the time, it was illegal in Washington. I was on the wrong side of the law for a while, but knowing that it helped me physically with my MS condition, I continued to get it.

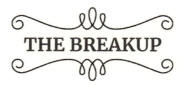
THE BREAKUP

When I was sixteen, I fell in love with a guy named Dwayne. While we were dating, I stumbled upon something terrible. It was an article in Reader's Digest, and it claimed that the average MS patient dies within ten years of diagnosis after going through a lot of physical problems. I read that I could go deaf, blind, and much more. I had made the heartwrenching decision that I loved Dwayne too much to destroy his life with such things.

So I lied to him.

I told him I was still in love with someone else. I didn't want to hurt him, but I didn't know of any other way to encourage him to get on with his life without me. The truth is, I never stopped loving him, and that love had just increased over the years, causing my heart to ache.

He was so upset when I told him the lie he cried, and it tore my heart out. I knew I had to stick with my decision and not destroy his life.

Weeks later, I was walking down Main street on the sidewalk when I heard a truck pull up behind me. I turned to look at who it was, and it was Dwayne. He said, "Get in." I did, and he started driving.

The silence was loud, and the tension was thick. Breaking the silence, he asked me, "Do you have a brain tumor?"

I chuckled and asked him, "Where did you hear that?"

He told me Susie (who was my cousin) had told him, but I didn't tell him that I had Multiple Sclerosis. I didn't say anything more to him about it, and he dropped me off. I knew he was trying to make sense out of our breakup.

Years went by, and Dwayne and my paths crossed continuously, but I hid my feelings, crying and dreaming of him. My mother convinced me to go out with his brother Mike on the chance that I may get to see Dwayne. Mike told me he loved me and wanted to marry me. I replied carefully, trying not to hurt his feelings but clearly let him know I was in love with Dwayne; his response was that I could learn to love him. I gave it some thought for a few days and realized if I did, it would keep me from thinking about Dwayne all the time. It would also get me out of the house because I was sick of my parents fighting. In the back of my mind, I also thought that I could get an annulment and be away from my parents and get my own place, but that didn't happen.

Mike and I were married in October of 1980, and I did care for him. We had been married a couple of years when I started getting sick all of the time. I went to Dr. Lamb's office, where a nurse took a pregnancy test. The nurse came back to the waiting room where I was sitting, and she informed me that the test was positive. She then asked me if I wanted to set up the pregnancy termination. I glared at her, stood up, and said, "This baby has a better chance of being healthy than I do," and stormed out of the office.

I threw up daily for seven months. I couldn't hold food down or even stand the smell of it. I was supposed to gain weight with her, but I ended up losing two pounds while pregnant. I had a boy's name picked out because I was just sure it would be a boy, and his name was supposed to be Michael Lee.

I delivered the baby by c-section because the umbilical cord was wrapped around my baby's shoulders and neck. With every contraction, the baby's heart would skip a beat. To my amazement, when I woke up from the anesthesia, Mike was standing over me and told me we had a girl! Since I didn't have a name picked out for her, Mike and I decided we would keep the same middle name since it was his cousin David's and my mom's middle name. We both liked the name, Chris and Christi. I had seen the name Christa on a continued story that I had been watching, so we chose Christa Lee for her name.

My love had only increased for Dwayne secretly, and my thoughts were consumed by him. So much that one night while sleeping, I said his name out loud. Mike didn't appreciate it. Three years into that marriage, we broke up, and I moved my daughter and me into a little apartment.

There, I met a woman named Sue, and we became best friends. She had a daughter, Bridget, who was one year older than my daughter. Christa was five and a half months old when her father and I separated.

Unfortunately, we made a few bad decisions together. Sue and I drank alcohol and snorted cocaine together. There was a vent in my living room that was joined to my landlord's apartment, which allowed my landlord to hear everything going on in my apartment. Sue and I had friends over one night, and because of the laughing and ruckus we caused all night, my landlord was beating on the door at 6 am the next morning. She was kicking us out, and we had to leave right away.

Sue had a friend named Jessie who took the two of us in with our daughters. Christa and I didn't live with Jessie very long because that summer, I stepped in a hole and sprained my ankle. My grandma Lola had found out and rode over in a taxi, packed our stuff, loaded us into the car, and took us home with her. We stayed with grandma Lola through the fall and winter. In the spring, I moved into a house with my boyfriend, Barry.

During this time, I was really clumsy, but I was still on my feet. I partied a lot and felt like a loser for doing so. My daughter started having convulsions, scaring me into being straight for a while. I kept running to the doctor with her every time she would have a seizure. The doctors never did give me any answers why it was happening. I knew Christa was running a fever during the episodes. All that the doctors would tell me is that she would grow out of it, and she did, thank God. But it was very scary, especially not knowing what was happening with my baby. Once I knew she was ok, I began to party again.

Barry was gone for days at a time, and he was extremely mean and destructive when he would come home drunk. One night, he didn't get home until really late. A friend of his, Rob, started beating on the front door less than an hour after Barry had come home. The door was near my daughter's bedroom. After the third time of Rob beating on the door, and I repeatedly told him to stop or he would wake up my daughter, I yanked open the door and punched him, causing Rob to roll off the front porch. After all the commotion, Barry got up and left with him anyway. Rob walked around the next day with a shiner, bragging that I gave it to him.

I became seriously addicted to cocaine, and I allowed my mother to raise my daughter the majority of the time. The MS seemed to be at a standstill, and I used cocaine for the energy level I lacked. The cocaine that I used for the energy didn't come without a price. The addiction was horrific, and the more I tried to get away from it, the more my body wanted.

I became someone I didn't want to be.

Sue and I began shooting up; cocaine became my world. The smell of ether and ringing in my ears was normal for me.

I had separated from Barry when I began to overdose fairly often. Kenny, my boyfriend at the time, and his brother Larry would get on each side of me and help me walk it off when I was so close to death. The cold, crisp air would help me to breathe again.

I wore long sleeve shirts to cover up the tracks even though it was so hot you couldn't breathe in the summer. I sold my furniture for cocaine, then I sold my stereo, my bed, and much more. When I ran out of things to sell for coke, I rented my mobile home to one of my dealers. He paid me with coke, and it was gone in one night. I lived on the streets for one month with Barry, who had come back into my life.

When I got so sick from not eating, drinking, and drugging, I showed up on my mother's doorstep. I was unable to stand up all the way because my stomach had shrunk so much, and my chest was sunk in. When my mom opened the door, she got tears in her eyes and welcomed me with open arms. She literally spoon-fed me until I regained my appetite and was able to feed myself. She took me shopping for clothes that would actually fit instead of hanging loosely on me. Mom took me to a 12-step meeting, Narcotics Anonymous, or "NA," where they surrounded me with support and helped me stay clean.

After I had been at my mom's house a couple of days and was lying in bed ready to go to sleep, my baby girl wanted to come to sleep with mommy. That night, withdrawals hit me so hard, and the pain was so intense in my stomach I was screaming in my mind with pain. I was ever so careful not to disturb my baby girl who was lying next to me.

My friends in NA and AA helped me overcome my mistakes by helping me get my home back. I had gotten into drugs so deeply that my daughter was almost taken from me. During the meetings, I was constantly reminded of the depth of my addiction. Once I got to where I could forgive myself for all the overdoses, I became very grateful to God that He kept me alive, and I was able to keep my daughter. Realizing God had brought me through so much, I turned my life back to Him.

I started modeling Under Cover Wear lingerie, taking advantage of the thin body that drugs had reduced me to. My friend Sue was also thin, so I talked her into modeling with me part-time. It was fun but embarrassing at times. We had shows in different towns, and they were easy, but shows at home where people knew me made it harder to be professional.

One show we did was a co-ed in a double-wide trailer, and as I made my second turn on the floor, my ex-boyfriend Kenny—who was seeing my friend Sue at the time—opened the drapes. When the natural light hit the gown I was wearing, it was no longer sparkling and shimmering, but it was see-through, and I ran off to the dressing room even though I knew it was unprofessional. From that moment on, the lighting had to be dim, or they could forget having me model! Because through it all, I was still modest to an extent.

Being straight and sober, the old me was back.

I came to the realization that instead of having my mother help raise my baby while I was being selfish and worrying about my own agenda, I needed to step up and be a full-time mom. Christa was all that was in my life; I loved her so much, focusing on her kept me grounded, and I was able to look forward to her future. All of her years growing up, I tried to teach her that the most important thing in life is to put God first.

My daughter grew up to marry her high school sweetheart, and they had three kids, so I have three grandkids to love and live for. They were a charge and kept me going, especially when I felt that giving up was an option. All of my life, I have stood on knowing that I could never give up, and the fight was constant.

MEDICATION FREE

My heart still ached for Dwayne, as I have always been in love with him. I needed to see him, so I paid my roommate to take me to his house in Wenatchee. He had no clue I was coming, and I crashed his party where he and his friends were playing cards. We stayed the night there, and the next morning, Dwayne mentioned the idea of raising our daughters together. I got so excited; I felt like my life was finally going to be alright.

My roommate and I left and went home. A short time later, I was raped by a truck driver heading to Canada. It really had an effect on the way I looked at life and messed with my mind, feeling like I brought it upon myself for breaking my promise that I would not destroy Dwayne's life with my inevitable future.

When Dwayne showed up at my house one day, he asked to go inside while I was outside. I had assumed he was going in to use the restroom after his long trip. I waited outside, thinking he would come back out to talk to me, but he must have expected me to follow him in. I should have followed him in because, when he finally did come out, he simply left without saying a word. I felt like that was the moment we could have talked about important things and our feelings for each other, but I blew it. We haven't spoken since then.

On a later date, I saw him with a cute hippy chick. I was with my mom, and when he saw us, he turned and walked away. I took that as a hint that he really didn't want to talk. I didn't blame him at all and hoped for his happiness. I know the chance of standing before God could happen at any time, and I can't stand before him without being honest with this man since my health has been deteriorating. I think what scared me the most was being afraid of never feeling the way I did when he held me. I have always kept everyone at arm's length, away from my heart, but for some reason, when he was holding me, that hard exterior would melt every time, scaring the crap out of me because I was breaking my own promise to myself. I love him; I always have and always will. I begged God to help me to never hurt him again by giving in and being a part of his life.

The man I ended up marrying was my friend at the time, Mike. We took that friendship to the next level, realizing I needed to look out for myself. We were like fire and gasoline, and it was a rocky relationship because of the obvious. I got into a relationship with Mike before I was really ready to move on.

Soon after we had gotten together, Mike sat Christa up on his lap and asked her what she thought about him asking me to marry him. Christa said, "I don't know, I'll think about it," in her 4-year-old voice. Christa jumped down and went to bed, leaving an awkward silence. I think Mike did that to break the ice with me because he knew how I felt about marriage at that point, knowing I had been married and divorced twice already. When he asked me to marry him, I caved and said yes, and we were married on November 19th, 1988.

My mobile home caught fire while we were gone one day. When we returned home, there were flames coming out of my skylight. We jumped out of the car. Mike ran to the front of the house, grabbed the hot doorknob, and opened it. When the air hit the fire, the flames exploded! I stood in the yard with Christa watching the fire, trying to keep her calm while she cried. Mike was panicked and wanted to save anything he could. He grabbed a couch pillow and threw it out the door, and that was the only thing he could save.

After the house was destroyed, we moved in with Mike's sister and her family on Mount Hull. I'm grateful for them taking us in, but it was the shits!

I let my daughter spend more time with my mom again since she was expected to do hard chores with Mike's nieces and nephew. She was still so young, and the chores she was expected to help with were too much for her, and that made me angry.

We moved into a shack that was not built properly by someone who didn't know what they were doing. When sitting on the couch, I could watch the deer graze in the yard between the boards on the wall. The winter was so cold that Mike had to put a tarp up on the outside of the house to try to hold the heat in. At night, I would put a stocking hat on Christa and pile quilts and blankets on her to keep her warm.

Our woodstove was literally glowing red, and you could still see your breath in the house. Mike had to be careful because the insulation started to glow around the stove pipe. Needless to say, that house was a fire hazard. We had an outhouse that we used, and we would have to bring the toilet seat inside with us and take it back out when we needed to use it. It was impossible to sit on when it was really cold outside.

One day, Mike and I got into a fight. He went to his sister's house, and I took off walking down the mountain—which I started to regret. It was 30 degrees below zero with the wind chill factor and a blizzard going on. Hypothermia was setting in when I ran into Mike's nieces and Christa, who were walking home from the school bus. I was already stiffening up, and the girls turned me around and helped me back to Mike's sister's house. I took my hat and scarf off and put them around my daughter since she had left hers on the bus.

We sat by Mike's sister's wood stove until he returned, then we were thawed out enough to go home.

As soon as we could, we moved back to town. We stayed at my mom's house until an apartment opened up. As Mike and I were walking past the school to go to a friend's funeral, his ex-girlfriend pulled up next to us on her bicycle. She informed Mike that his daughter would like to get to know him. We were shocked because she had told Mike years before that she had lost the baby.

An apartment opened up soon after, and it happened to be in the same complex as was Mike's daughter and her family. She became part of our lives for years until she decided to not come around anymore.

By this time, I was in the process of buying my own home. It was a cute three-bedroom, two-bath home. Mike was working construction, so we were no longer dirt poor. We opened an art gallery called "Useable Art

Gallery" with Dave and Jeff. We would have dinner parties at our house with other business owners. Our lives had changed drastically, and I was now living the way I wanted to live. Rubbing elbows with other business owners, we became pillars of our community.

My husband and I met with a group of our friends and went to the Sandpoil River to fish. We camped at a campground on the reservation while everyone except me went Walleye fishing. I sat on the lawn outside of our tent, nauseated and hurting and feeling like I was going to throw up. I couldn't take my medicine on an empty stomach, and I was too sick to eat. I cried out to God, *what should I do?* I heard a Still Small Voice that said, "Stop taking them." So, that handful of pills went back into the bottle, and I stopped taking all medication.

Amazingly, I got better.

Sometimes, medication isn't the answer. I

don't want to discourage anyone from taking medication that is working for them. I just know that the medication wasn't right for me; God let me know that. I left that camping trip with an ice chest of Walleye and felt incredible.

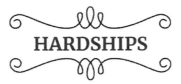

HARDSHIPS

When my daughter was in her teens, we had seven kids living with us. Some of them had been homeless, and some needed a place to stay for just a little while. The youngest kid staying with us had a heart condition and was left on the mountain to fend for himself. We took them all in with no financial help whatsoever, and we didn't care because they needed us.

As time went by, the kids moved away. Christa and her friend Segornae were the only ones left in the house. When they turned seventeen, they both ended up with decent vehicles and good jobs. Christa worked at the Canadian border, and Segornae worked at the nursing home. The girls approached me with the idea of them getting an apartment together, and they convinced me they could take care of themselves and pay bills, so I agreed.

After being in that house for more than eleven years, I received a letter saying they were going to increase my house payments to an amount that exceeded what I made in a month. Mike and I decided to sell the house and buy property.

It was twenty acres, we had a water-well put in, and we were in the process of putting electricity in when president Obama announced electricity would go up 80%. We lived off the grid for eight years before moving back to town. During the years that we lived up there, the hardships were tremendous, especially during winters.

While looking for natural remedies, I saw a video about Rick Simpsons oil.

I used it twice a day and began to regain strength.

My sister-in-law made comments to us about the oil because it contained marijuana, which was still illegal at the time. Mike and I knew she would jump at the chance of turning us in, even though it was helping us, so we quit taking it. Right after we quit taking the oil, my gallbladder started giving me a lot of trouble, so my diet had to change.

While living up there on the property, we had up to seven horses at one time. The horses we had were great therapy. Mine her was named Lakota; she was very well trained with an awesome temperament.

I looked everywhere for a disabled saddle so that I could ride her, but I never found one. I found myself daydreaming out the window a lot, watching the horses run down the hill with their mane and tail blowing in the wind so gracefully, wishing I was on their backs.

In addition to the horses, we also had chickens, rabbits, and a turkey. We raised hogs, too—mostly Yorkshire and Duroc. A farm is what it was, and I never imagined myself living on a farm.

The summers were nice on the hill because the thermal winds kept it cool. The winters were hard when the water lines would break, and Mike had to dig down through snow and ice, searching for the break.

One day, my heart started acting up, and we had to call an ambulance. It took an hour for them to get up our driveway. They still couldn't even get all the way up to the house, so the EMTs carried me to the ambulance.

Recently, I had lost my parents and many other family members and friends, which caused depression to set in.

My baby sister Tammy had beautiful, long, dark red hair, and she was always looking up to me for guidance and advice. We were very close. My sister died at a young age, which caused me to fight a deep depression, even more than I ever had to deal with in years. I realized it was taking my health down, so I had to pull myself out of it. I kept praying for a change in my life to happen when I received a letter in the mail stating that the state was going to take my mother's house. I called the Attorney General's office to see if there was a chance I could make payments to get the house out of jeopardy of being lost. Since I was disabled, they told me that the house was mine and they would forgive my mother's debt.

I went to see a lawyer to get the house put in my name for tax purposes. My husband and I moved off the mountain and into the house. I felt safer now with utilities and a roof over my head.

Mike and I separated, but he came back from what I felt was an obligation to help me since I did not have any caregivers and I was using a wheelchair full time. Mike and I had become more like good friends by then. He would come to my house and care for me.

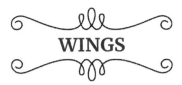
WINGS

My bladder totally stopped working, forcing me to get a surgery where they placed an unsightly tube into my bladder (super pubic catheter). I'm just now beginning to accept it— emotionally and mentally—as it's part of me now. Looking at the bright side of everything, I don't have to jump up and pee every few minutes. If you can, always look at the bright side, am I right?!

It's finally warming up outside to get out, but right now, that's not a good idea. The

Coronavirus pandemic has swept through our state putting people with weak immune systems at risk. So, I stay inside trying to stay healthy, and I take immune builders.

My daughter and grandchildren lived with me, and they did their best to not get me sick and bring it to me. Isolating seems like the only way to stop this thing. The schools shut down; therefore, my grandchildren were home all the time. They were getting bored from being shut-in, and I'll be glad when this virus blows over.

My energy is bottled up, and I need an outlet. So, I decided to write this book to share my advice for anyone with MS.

The most important thing is to be positive in all situations and to not lose sight of your dreams. There is no expiration date stamped on the bottom of our feet. Do not take the word of doctors telling you that you aren't going to live or articles that give you no hope. Be positive and look at the bright side of everything, and don't let anyone bring you down. I've had MS for quite a few years now and have no plans of leaving this earth yet.

Genuine friends are so important, and the support system is crucial.

Being in a wheelchair can be your wings when you can't move or can be your anchor, feeling like you can't do anything anymore. I choose wings continuously, having a good outlook on life.

Throughout my life, I have seen so many doctors that I never remember them all, and I've tried every prescription for my MS they come up with. The prescriptions made me sick every time, yet I would still try them in hopes that they found something that would work.

Throughout the years of having MS, I've had many care providers come and go, some good, some bad. I have finally found a couple of young ladies that I think will stick. I deeply love them both and their families. In fact, they are helping me write this book by giving wings to my fingers. (Thank you, girls.)

I am grateful for their help because I no longer have the ability to stand at this point. For now, I have to be moved from my bed to my wheelchair, then I have freedom again.

I spend little time alone because of my inabilities right now, but the rare time I am alone, I spend it thinking about the young man I fell in love with when I was a teenager, wishing I could apologize to him for all the times I left him confused. It was never about him. I wish I had had a chance to tell him that.

Dwayne, the man I was so in love with, who is a major part of my story, had passed away from cancer. Rest in peace, Dwayne.

A piece of advice: live your life to its fullest. Eat a good diet, exercise continually, and look at the bright side of everything. Never let anyone tell you there is a time limit on your life because only God knows when your time is. My motto is to never give up!

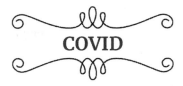
COVID

After not contracting COVID for quite some time, Mike, my caregivers, and I came down with it.

Mike had a heart attack while infected with Covid. My caregivers were sick with it, so therefore I had no help. Mike, as sick as he was, put couch cushions on my bedroom floor, making a bed for himself. He unselfishly slept in my room to watch over me because I was having a hard time breathing, which helped me watch him too. I realized at that point that we really do still love each other. And I've come to realize we don't die until God is ready for us!

My daughter had gotten a good job in Spokane, Washington, at Sacred Heart hospital. My daughter and the youngest grandchildren moved to Spokane. My oldest grandson just graduated from boot camp. He's a Marine now. It seems like yesterday he was making peanut butter cookies with Grandma. I'm praying for his safety daily, around the clock.

MRIs that I've had in the past have shown the lesions on my brain growing. When I was taking Rick Simpson's oil regularly, the scans began to show the lesions were shrinking. Since I haven't taken it for so long now, the headaches have worsened, which means they probably are growing more. The gadolinium, in contrast, caused my quick descent into the wheelchair, so I have no desire to take any more MRIs.

It is what it is.

I move from my bed to the chair using a Hoyer lift. The pain in the right frontal lobes of my brain and my inner ear feels like an ice pick stabbing in my head fairly often. I try not to take pain medications as much as possible because I don't like the way they make me feel. I definitely don't need another addiction.

Fifty-nine years of a totally eventful life, and I'm still not going anywhere.

I have three caregivers that I depend on for almost everything now. Multiple Sclerosis laying claims on my body at such a young age wasn't painful in my younger years; it just made me embarrassingly clumsy. I think the hardest thing for me to accept was when my oxygen levels lessened and my voice began to crack, causing me to not be able to hold a note when I sang. Singing was such a large part of my life, so losing that ability changed my life drastically. I've learned that looking on the bright side of everything is the only way to be. That attitude has helped me to overcome obstacles throughout the years.

I'm so overjoyed to be able to tell my story, and it has definitely not come to an end yet. I hope it will give you hope and help you through your life's obstacles.

Never, ever give up.

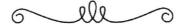

ABOUT THE AUTHOR

Tangie Essary was born in Tonasket, Washington. She has lived in Alaska, Arizona, and Montana but spent the majority of her life in Oroville, Washington.

Tangie was diagnosed with Multiple Sclerosis at the age of thirteen. Throughout her life, she has lived a beautiful, colorful life by teaching herself new skills to overcome the challenges of her condition.

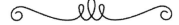

Made in the USA
Middletown, DE
17 September 2025